IT'S YOUR LIFE – AVOID THE COCKTAIL EFFECT OF HARMFUL CHEMICALS IN YOUR BODY

Professor Norman Ratcliffe

*A catalogue record for this book is available
from the British Library*

ISBN: 978-1-907962-58-5

Published by Cranmore Publications

www.cranmorepublications.co.uk

This book is dedicated to my parents whose undying faith in my academic capabilities allowed me to pursue a scientific career. My gratitude also goes to my sister, Teri King, whose success as an author and constant encouragement and advice were such sources of inspiration. Thanks too to my many friends for tolerating so many mealtime discussions on health and diet as well as the unsolicited advice given to them!

Finally, I wish to thank Dr. Duncan McLaren of Swansea Metropolitan University for his outstanding enthusiasm and imagination during creation of sections of this book as well as Doreen Montgomery of Rupert Crew Ltd for her patient and helpful comments of the manuscript.

"IT'S YOUR LIFE"

THE AUTHOR

- **Professor Norman Ratcliffe** is a founder member of a team that recently discovered a new antibiotic potentially capable of curing MRSA and *Clostridium difficile*. This work was presented to Prince Phillip at St. James's Palace, London and was the subject of major media attention in the UK on ITV News and in many leading newspapers, including the Wall Street Journal, around the World. He is a Fellow of the Royal Society of Medicine and has previously run a "Health Alert" blood-testing company. He has published over 200 books and research papers on immunology, cancer invasion, influenza, tropical diseases and MRSA. He played squash for Wales, ran the London Marathon at the age of 50 and works-out regularly in the gym.

- **Professor Ratcliffe** retired recently after 25 years as a University Research Professor. He decided to finally complete "It's Your Life" after 5 years work in order to help the many people who are confused about health and fitness issues and who have constantly been asking his advice.

"IT'S YOUR LIFE"

THE SERIES

Professor Norman Ratcliffe's comprehensive book on health is: *It's Your Life: End the confusion from inconsistent health advice:*

www.cranmorepublications.co.uk/6

This book will often be referred to as IYL. Alongside this comprehensive book there is a series of smaller *It's Your Life: End the confusion from inconsistent health advice* books; this book is the third in the series. The aim of the series is to give advice to people in specific areas; all of the areas covered in the series are also included in IYL. The series is as follows:

It's Your Life – A Healthy Diet Made Easy

www.cranmorepublications.co.uk/61

It's Your Life – Avoiding Harmful Chemicals in Your Food

www.cranmorepublications.co.uk/62

It's Your Life – Avoid the Cocktail Effect of Harmful Chemicals in Your Body

www.cranmorepublications.co.uk/63

It's Your Life – Vitamins and Supplements For All Ages

www.cranmorepublications.co.uk/64

It's Your Life – Exercise For All Ages

www.cranmorepublications.co.uk/65

The main advice arising from IYL has also been summarised in:

117 Health Tips: A quick guide for a healthy life

www.cranmorepublications.co.uk/7

Contents

THE COCKTAIL EFFECT

OH NO, NOT MORE CHEMICALS!

What is the Total Chemical Load of the Body from ALL SOURCES?

How to Reduce your Body Burden of Chemicals

All Parents Should Read This Book Since Babies And Children Are Potentially More Vulnerable Than Adults to Toxic Chemicals

If you just want to know how to avoid the most harmful chemicals present in the environment and how to reduce your "Body Burden" of chemicals then just read Section 5, which starts on page 55

In **It's Your Life – Avoiding Harmful Chemicals in Your Food** (Chapters 4 and 5 of IYL) it has been shown that our bodies are exposed to a large number of chemicals added artificially to our food and drink. In the present book, we reveal additional, potentially toxic chemicals, to which we are exposed to daily from numerous other sources including cosmetics and furnishings.

Figure 1. Shows the origin of the many chemicals that we are exposed to and which form a cocktail in the body

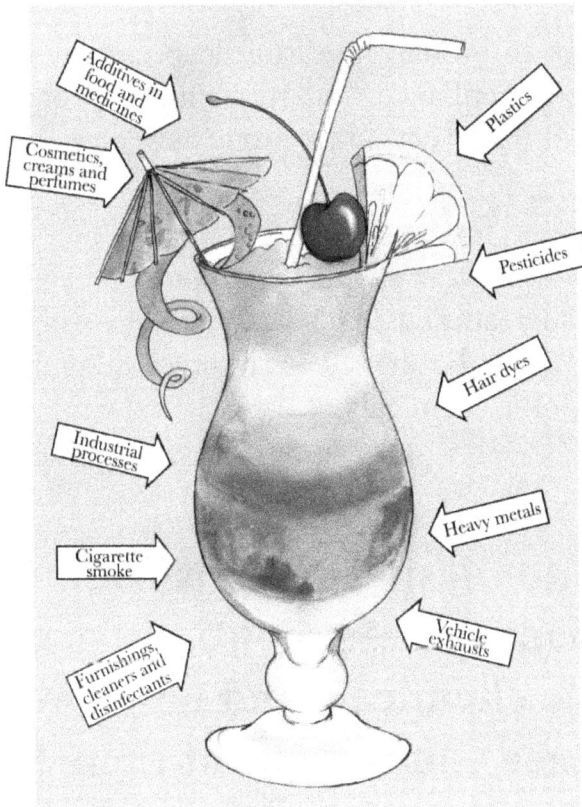

THERE IS NO ESCAPE FROM THESE CHEMICALS

Except to go and live in a deep cave with no modern appliances or furnishings, processed food, drink or consumer products.

In addition, few people have the time or know-how to read and understand minute labels on food, drink, cosmetics etc in order to avoid the most toxic chemicals.

Do not despair as this book will identify the potentially most toxic chemicals and help you to reduce your intake of these (see Sections 1 and 5, below).

According to the **World Wildlife Fund** our environment is becoming increasingly contaminated by industrial chemicals, most of which have not been tested for their potential risk to human health (see reference 41).

In addition, we are exposed to a vast array of chemicals from consumer goods. For example, an **Environmental Working Group (EWG)** (www.ewg.org/reports) study showed that "89 percent of 10,500 ingredients used in personal care products have not been evaluated for safety by any publicly accountable institution."

The end result is that our bodies contain a mixture of these chemicals called, the **"BODY BURDEN"**. These chemicals are taken up via our food and drink and through the skin and lungs, and they may interact to magnify their harmful effect on the body and this process is called

"THE COCKTAIL EFFECT"

It is common sense to reduce the numbers of chemicals taken in, as **nobody** knows their long-term cumulative effect, i.e. **"The Cocktail Effect"**, on our health.

A major problem is that although organisations (such as the Food Standards Agency in the UK) set limits on levels of chemicals, including pesticides and additives, they ONLY usually consider individual chemicals on their own. UNFORTUNATELY, mixtures of additives are found in many products and these may accumulate and interact in the body to greatly magnify their toxicity/side effects (See, Section 3, "Synergistic Effects", below).

- **This book deals with:**

1. Sources of chemicals that we are exposed to and which are potentially most toxic

2. The "Body Burden" of these chemicals and which are most commonly found in the tissues of the body

3. Evidence for a synergistic (i.e. interactive) effect of these chemicals

4. Possible harmful effects of the "Body Burden" of chemicals and their link to disease

5. Avoidance/reduction of "Body Burden" of chemicals and strategies for detoxification (detox)

SECTION 1: SOURCES OF CHEMICALS TAKEN INTO THE BODY

The following Table 1 identifies the sources and chemicals of some concern. For additional details, the reader should consult the websites for the **Environmental Working Group (EWG)** (see reference 42), and also for the **World Wildlife Fund** (see reference 41).

Table 1.   SOURCES OF ARTIFICIAL CHEMICALS OF PARTICULAR   SAFETY CONCERNS INCLUDED IN "THE COCKTAIL EFFECT"

Source of Chemical	Name of Chemical	Safety Concerns and Possible Health Effects
i. Pesticides In food and drink	**Persistent Organic Pollutants (POPs).** Include DDT, HCH and aldrin	**POPs** may cause breast and other cancers, suppress the immune system, disturb hormonal functions and fertility, and pollute human breast milk with short and long-term consequences. Not all POPs are pesticides eg. PCBs and dioxins (see xi. and xii., below).
ii. Additives In food, drink and medicines	**Colourants, preserva-tives, sweeteners etc.** Includes azo dyes, benzoates, sulphites, aspartame	Some **additives** may be involved in cancer formation, behavioural/learning problems in children, as well as the aggravation of allergies and hypersensitivity, and the induction of organ damage through oxidative stress and weight gain.

| iii. Some cosmetics and makeup, lipstick, moisterizers, suncreams, deodorants, hairsprays, shampoos, perfumes, shaving cream and even in toddlers toothpaste contain mixtures of potentially toxic chemicals | **Parabens** (methyl- ,ethyl-, propyl- and butyl- parabens) | **Parabens** are preservatives and have also been approved for use in food and medicines (= E214-219) as well as cosmetics for many years (see reference 43). Parabens are present in human breast cancer tissue. They can mimic the female sex hormone, oestrogen, which has been linked to breast cancer as well as the disruption of sperm production in rats (see reference 44). Parabens can also cause rashes and skin allergies. Parabens may accumulate in women with long term use of cosmetics, particularly of under arm deodorants/perfumes. The FDA[1] and cosmetics producers view is that parabens in cosmetics are safe due to the low levels used BUT neither the "long term accumulation effect" nor the "cocktail effect" have been tested in detail. |

| iv. Some cosmetics and makeup, lipstick, moisterizers, suncreams, deodorants, hairsprays, shampoos, perfumes, shaving creams and even toddlers toothpaste contain mixtures of potentially toxic chemicals | Polyethylene glycols (PEGs) Contaminated with ethylene dioxide, 1,4-dioxane and polycyclic aromatic hydrocarbons (PAH) | PEGs keep the ingredients of the cosmetic mixed and help spreading over the skin. Generally, PEGs are regarded as safe although safety tests are incomplete (see reference 45). The main problem is with the contaminants in PEGs. They may contain various harmful impurities including: **Ethylene oxide** which increases the incidences of uterine and breast cancers and of leukemia and brain cancer. **1, 4-dioxane** which according to the US EPA[2] is a "probable human carcinogen" and also causes irritation to the eyes, nose, throat, lungs and skin as well as liver and kidney damage. **Polycyclic aromatic compounds** (PAHs) which are known to increase the risk of breast cancer. |
| v. Some cosmetics etc, as above, for Parabens and PEGs | Propylene glycol | **Popylene glycol** is present in many cosmetics, moisturisers, shampoos, foods and medicines. Regarded as safe in food but may cause allergic reactions in skin (dermatitis) and lungs, irritates the eyes, penetrates the skin and may cause kidney or liver damage. |

| vi. Common in shampoos, soaps, bubble bath, shower gels, shaving foam, washing up liquid, toothpaste, carpet and floor cleaners, car wash. | Sodium lauryl sulphate (SLS or SDS) | **SLS** is a strong detergent/lathering agent and present in over 75% of shampoos and conditioners. It is **highly irritating to the skin in some people** and can trigger dermatitis. The Data Safety Sheet for SLS[3] states "avoid contact with skin and eyes", mutagenic (may cause cancer), may accumulate in the body and cause organ damage, if inhaled get medical attention immediately (!). Also, found in children's products! |
| vii. Some food, hairsprays, deodorants, nail polish, perfumes, suncreams, table cloths, floor tiles, furnishings, shower curtains, rainwear, dolls, some toys, car upholstery, | Phthalates (eg. DBP and DEHP) | **Phthalates** are added to plastics to make them more flexible and are widely distributed in the environment from factories, leaching from plastic in landfill sites or from burning. They are also released indoors from plastic products. Phthalates have been detected in the blood and urine of most people tested. Phthlataes are hormone disruptors and may increase both the risk of birth defects and reproductive abnormalities as well as breast cancer in women. Exposure to |

food packaging, plastic water bottles.		low levels of phthalates may occur from beauty products, by eating food in plastic packages, by breathing dust in rooms with furnishings and by drinking bottled water, all of which may contain phthalates. Some phthalates are banned by European Union from children's soft toys, teething rings and dummies[4]- beware some imports!
viii. In polycarbon-ate plastics for baby and water bottles, sports equipment, dental fillings, and electronics. Epoxy resins with bisphenol A used to coat the inside of food and drink cans. Bisphenol is also a flame retardant	**Bisphenol A (BPA)**	**Bisphenol A** is used in a wide range of plastics but most concern is with it's **presence in baby bottles and linings of cans** from which it may leach into food and drink. The FSA[5], the EFSA[6] and the FDA[1] all believe that the amount of BPA to which babies and children are being exposed does "not indicate a safety concern" and is "without appreciable risk". Unfortunately, like phthalates, BPA is another hormone disruptor in animal studies but controversy surrounds the risk of BPA to humans, due to limited studies. The NTP[7] stated that "several studies collectively suggest hormonal effects in humans". With

precursor.		mounting public concern, Canada and several USA States are banning the sale/importation of polycarbonate baby bottles.
ix. Sunscreen, facial moisturisers, lipsticks and lip balm.	**Oxybenzone** = Benzophenone-3	**Oxybenzone** is present in over 40% of sunscreens. It is readily absorbed through the skin and may cause hormone disruption and low birth weight of girls[8]. Much more data required but caution worthwhile.
x. In soft furnishings eg. in foam cushions, mattresses, as well as children's pyjamas, plastics of TVs and computers.	**Flame retardants (eg. polybrominated diphenyl ethers= PBDE)**	**Like pesticides (above), PBDEs are POPs (see i. Pesticides, above)** and enter and persist in the environment and pass up the food chain to be eaten and accumulate in human fat. They then enter human breast milk and pass into the foetus and baby. They are present throughout the environment, in air, water and food, and are impossible to avoid. In mice, they are toxic to the liver, thyroid, and are also neurotoxins and endocrine disruptors. They are banned by the EU but continue to accumulate in landfill sites from old furniture foam and electronics plastic.

| xi. Previously, widely used in paints, adhesives, plastics, flame retardants, rubber and electrical goods eg. fluorescent lights. Coolants and lubricants in large electrical equipment – transformers capacitors etc. | Polychlorinated biphenyls (PCBs).

 Include over 100 different compounds. | PCBs are another group of Persistent Organic Pollutants POPs (see i. Pesticides, above). Despite the banning of PCBs and other POPS in many countries[9], they are still being found in human tissues. This is due to bioconcentration in food chains, through long-term environmental contamination of soils, water and air by industrial and incineration processes. As humans are at the top of many food chains we may ingest high levels of these POPs from fish, meat etc. These residual POPs may cause breast and other cancers, suppress the immune system, disturb hormonal functions and pollute breast milk with unknown short and long-term consequences for babies and infants. |

| xii. Produced by paper mills, waste incinerators etc, from cigarettes and exhausts. Most dioxins are ingested via full fat dairy produce and meat from animals fed on polluted pastures or feed. Dioxins dissolve in body fat and milk. Also, in poultry, eggs, cereals, fish and fish oils, and unwashed fruit and vegetables. | **Dioxins.** Include a group of about 17 chlorine-containing compounds. | **Dioxins are another group of Persistent Organic Pollutants POPs (see i. Pesticides, and xi. PCBs, above).** They are unintentional products from industry as well as from grass fires, volcanic activity etc. and are found throughout the environment in soils, water and air. They bioaccumulate in food chains into the human diet. The long-term effects, like the PCBs, probably involve the immune system, reproduction and development, including possible hormonal disturbances. Dioxins are also involved in a skin disease called chloracne with widespread pustules over the body. There are strong indications of increased risk of cancers in particular regions of the body and of the cancer-forming potential of dioxins. **The Seveso disaster released high levels of dioxins into adjacent areas and 10 years after the explosion, people were more likely to have cancer**[10]. Like PCBs and other POPs, dioxins are subject to the Stockholm Convention (2001)[9] and countries are obliged to take measures to eliminate and minimise all sources of dioxins.. |

1. FDA = Food and Drug Administration, USA
   (**www.fda.gov › Cosmetics**)

2. US EPA = United States Environmental Protection Agency
   (**www.epa.gov/ttnatw01/hlthef/dioxane.html**)

3. Material Safety Data Sheet for sodium lauryl sulphate
   (**www.sciencelab.com/xMSDS-Sodium_lauryl_sulfate-9925002**)

4. The Environment Agency

   (**www.environment-agency.gov.uk/business/39127.aspx**)

5. FSA = Food Standards Agency
   (**www.fsascience.net/2008/05/06/baby_bottle_safety**)

6. EFSA = European Food Safety Authority
   (**www.efsa.europa.eu/EFSA/efsa_locale-**

   1178620753812_1178710289744.htm)

7. The NTP = National Toxicology Program
   (**www.niehs.nih.gov/health/docs/bpa-factsheet.pdf**)

8. **www.medpagetoday.com/Dermatology/8927**

9. Stockholm Convention on Persistent Organic Pollutants, Stockholm,
   22 May 2001,

   (**www.pops.int/documents/signature/signstatus.htm**)

10. See reference 46

SECTION 2: THE "BODY BURDEN" OF CHEMICALS AND THOSE MOST COMMONLY PRESENT IN THE TISSUES

Table 1 (above), only lists **some** of the **most likely**, potentially toxic, chemicals that we may be exposed to. It does not include hair dyes, Teflon coatings (perfluorinated compounds, PFCs) of cooking pans, heavy metals such a tin, lead and mercury, or any of the other thousands of other chemicals registered with the EU.

Many of these chemicals will be broken down by the liver while others will remain and accumulate in the body for many years to form the **Body Burden.**

ALTHOUGH IT IS DIFFICULT TO PROVE BEYOND DOUBT, it is reasonable to assume that, after a certain point, the Body Burden may become toxic and contribute to disease (see, Section 4, below).

- **It is also most important to understand that foetuses in the womb, babies and rapidly developing children are likely to be more sensitive to chemical contaminants than are adults.**

- For example, **thyroid hormones (eg. thyroxine)** play key roles in foetal brain development, and contaminants, such as PCBs, may decrease thyroxine levels and disrupt normal foetal brain development.

- These contaminants **can be passed on to the foetus** and baby via the mother's milk at all stages of development. They can also adversely affect the foetus **well below** levels described as "safe" in the adult woman.

Avoid the cocktail effect

Of the 12 groups of chemicals listed in Table 1 (above), it is important to know which ones accumulate in the body and therefore could potentially by themselves, or by interacting with others, over time, produce disease.

A number of **BIOMONITORING STUDIES (= tests on body tissues over several years)** have been or are being carried out to detect the presence and levels of chemical contaminants in the blood, urine, fat, breast milk and other tissues of people.

One of the largest studies is the Canadian Health Measures Survey of 5,000 volunteers using biomonitoring tests for 60 chemicals and heavy metals which is being carried out over a number of cycles beginning in 2007 and continuing into 2011 and beyond (see reference 47).

Other studies by the Centers for Disease Control (USA) Biomonitoring and Body Burden Reports are also ongoing. Report Number 3, 2005, measured 148 chemicals in the blood or urine collected from 2,400 people. It showed in the USA that levels of some harmful substances, including lead, dioxin, DDT and mercury, were declining. On the other hand, phthalate levels (from plastics) generally remained the same over several years with higher levels in women and 6-11 year old children (see reference 48).

In addition, other studies of human **Body Burdens** have identified contaminant chemicals remaining in the tissues where they can potentially cause harm. These studies include:

1. The World Wildlife Fund (WWF) – UK, National Biomonitoring Survey, 2003 (see reference 49)

2. The Environmental Working Group, Human Toxome Project, 2007 (see reference 50)

1. **The WWF Survey (UK)** analysed human blood serum from 155 volunteers, all of whom were 18yr or older, for levels of contaminant chemicals. A large range of well-known Persistent Organic Pollutants (POPs) were tested for including PCBs, pesticides and flame retardants (see Table 1). **The results showed that the people had, on average, 27 different chemicals in their blood** and that:

- PCBs were commonly present but levels were significantly lower than in previous surveys.

- DDT and HCH were the predominant pesticides present but their levels too were significantly lower than in previous surveys.

- There was widespread presence of the PBDE flame retardants.

- The source of the PCBs and pesticides was thought to be food while the flame retardants may have been from house dust.

2. In the Environmental Working Group, Human Toxome Project, 2007, up to 532 different contaminant chemicals were tested for in the blood, urine, or breast milk of 174 American people from babies in the uterus or newborn, teens, adults and seniors (over 65 yr) and:

- The chemicals detected included many of those described in Table 1 (above) such as pesticides, parabens, PAHs, bisphenol, PBDE, PCBs and dioxins, as well as many other contaminants including PFCs, lead, mercury etc. The presence of dioxins, mercury, PFCs and PCBs in the newborns is of concern.

In conclusion, we have a good indication that many groups of chemical contaminants find their way into the human body where they may remain and could potentially contribute to disease.

SECTION 3: EVIDENCE FOR A SYNERGISTIC (i.e. INTERACTIVE) EFFECT OF THESE CHEMICALS ON THE BODY

This section discusses opposing scientific views of synergism so if you just wish to know the basic conclusions go to page 48 and Section 5, below.

Studies **are extremely difficult to design** to test for the possible increase in toxicity of contaminants resulting from their interaction in the body with each other, i.e. **the Cocktail Effect.** This is because:

i. Mixtures of contaminants present in the environment vary greatly and also vary between different populations of people. For example, rural versus city dwellers or babies versus senior citizens will be exposed to differing cocktails of chemicals in their food and air (see reference 50).

ii. Any interactions between contaminants would be complex since the chemicals may have different targets in the body, may be broken down or stored differently and may activate or inhibit each other.

iii. We know from biomonitoring (see Section 2, above) that mixtures of contaminants commonly occur in people. However, most reports on the effects of mixtures of chemical come from studies on animals or from laboratory experiments. Information on humans is limited as experiments with people are strictly controlled.

iv. Finally, levels of contaminants in mixtures are often very low, making assessment of their impact even more difficult.

OPINIONS ABOUT THE COCKTAIL EFFECT USUALLY FALL INTO ONE OF TWO CONTRASTING GROUPS:

1. The official "independent Government" opinion represented by the Food Standards Agency (FSA). This agency confirms that there is evidence for exposure of people to mixtures of chemicals but concludes that **there is only limited evidence for any adverse effects of such combinations** (see references 51, 52).

2. Many other groups, that are independent of governments and supported by members, including the World Wildlife Fund (WWF)-UK (www.wwf.org.uk), the Environmental Working Group (EWG) (www.ewg.org), and the Pesticide

Action Network (PAN) (www.pan-uk.org), believe that **the cocktail effect is extremely serious and urgent action is required.**

SO WHO SHOULD YOU BELIEVE?

- The Food Standards Agency (FSA) commissioned a report by the Committee on Toxicity on a "Risk Assessment of Mixtures of Pesticides and Similar Substances". This 2002 report, was extremely detailed, nearly 300 pages long, and considered all aspects of risks from chemical mixes. It reviewed previous scientific papers on the toxic effects of chemical mixtures, mainly pesticides and veterinary medicines. In most cases, **it was concluded that there was, for one reason or another, very little evidence for enhanced effects of mixtures** (see references 51, 52).

This report was produced by extremely well-qualified scientists although the links that some members had with chemical/pharmaceutical companies are noted.

- The FSA's view seems to coincide with that of the American Chemistry Council (ACC) who pointed out that each day, as we breathe air or eat, our bodies absorb a mixture of low level natural and man-made chemicals (see reference 53). All life's activities are fuelled by chemical reactions and therefore it is not surprising that as the sensitivity of biomonitoring increases more and more chemicals will be detected at lower and lower concentrations. The potential for harm or toxicity will be determined very much by **the dose and exposure time** of these chemicals. Even natural chemicals can be toxic at high enough doses but most chemicals can be dealt with by the body at low doses. **The ACC therefore**

believes that we must not be too concerned about these low dose mixtures of chemicals.

• However, the opposing view of the WWF, EWG and PAN, **that even at low levels, individual or cocktails of chemicals are potentially harmful**, has some significant supporting evidence. For example:

i. WWF points out that **there is very good evidence from wildlife to show just how harmful some of these contaminants, including pesticides, can be.** Even at low levels in the blood, they can accumulate in the fat tissues. For example, there are many accounts that the pesticide, DDT, resulted in the thinning of the eggshells of birds of prey (although this is disputed) and subsequent declines in populations of these birds in the UK, and that PCBs have seriously affected seal immunity (see reference 54). Both of these chemicals accumulate in humans too (see Biomonitoring in Section 2, above). Ok, this is not evidence for chemical interaction in a cocktail but illustrates that low levels of contaminants accumulate in tissues and may be harmful.

SO WHY SHOULD THERE NOT ALSO BE AN EFFCT IN HUMANS, NOT JUST FROM THESE TWO BANNED CHEMICALS, BUT FROM OTHERS ACCUMULATING SINGLY OR IN MIXTURES TOO?

ii. There are now also more recent reports, since the FSA study in 2002, supporting the idea that cocktails of chemicals can interact and have enhanced toxic effects.

- For example, it has been shown in the laboratory that **combinations of commonly used food additives are much more toxic when added to mouse nerve cells than what would be expected from the sum of the toxicity of the individual food additives.** This synergistic toxic effect represents about a 3 fold increase in toxicity than expected just from the toxicity of the individual additives added together. The combinations of additives used showing this synergistic toxic (interactive) effect were monosodium glutamate, brilliant blue and aspartame with quinoline yellow (see Chapter 5 of IYL, Tables 1 and 3). The doses of additives used were about the same as would occur in the blood after a child had a snack and a drink (see reference 55).

- **Another simpler example of chemical interaction resulted from the discovery of the cancer–forming chemical, benzene, in soft drinks.** The benzene resulted from the interaction of the preservative, sodium benzoate, with vitamin C in the drinks. A FSA survey showed that about 30% of 150 soft drinks tested in the UK contained benzene and levels were sufficiently high to result in removal of 4 of these from sale (see reference 56). This example is important as it shows an interaction between a potential toxin, sodium benzoate, with a safe vitamin to produce a totally unexpected highly carcinogenic substance, benzene. What other surprises await discovery in chemical cocktails?

- **There are many other examples of the cocktail effect including studies on wildlife of mixtures of chemicals found in aquatic habitats.** Thus, exposure of salmon to mixtures of organophosphate and carbamate pesticides, which are commonly found in rivers, resulted in significantly higher levels of brain enzyme damage than would be expected just by addition of the toxicity of the two individual pesticides alone (see reference 57). The levels of pesticides used were similar to those found in the natural habitats of salmon. These results are relevant to mammals, too, as they have the same brain enzymes targeted by the pesticides above.

CONCLUSION

REDUCE YOUR BODY BURDEN OF CHEMICALS

Since evidence is now increasing indicating that:

- Low levels of contaminants can accumulate in tissues of the body and then cause toxic effects

- Contaminants can sometimes produce significantly higher levels of toxicity in combinations than that resulting from simple addition of the toxicity of the chemicals used alone. For example, if 10% of animals were killed by each chemical used by itself then when two were used in combination killing was not 20% but 50% or more i.e. a 30% Cocktail Effect

SECTION 4: POSSIBLE HARMFUL EFFECTS OF THE "BODY BURDEN" OF CHEMICALS AND THEIR LINK TO ONSET OF DISEASE

- In most Western countries, the incidences of breast, testicular and prostate cancer, asthma, allergies, birth defects, low sperm counts, early puberty, behavioural and learning problems, cardiovascular disease, obesity and diabetes are on the increase.

- No doubt some, but not all, of these increases have resulted from improvements in diagnostic techniques and from various national campaigns to enhance screening for breast, prostate and bowel cancers.

- Other factors, however, must be accounting for some of these increases in human disease since conditions, such as breast cancer and testicular cancer, have doubled in the UK since 1984 and 1975, respectively (see reference 58).

- In addition, over the last 20 years, the incidence of allergic disease has increased dramatically worldwide. In England alone, anaphylaxis (extremely rapid and dangerous allergic reaction to peanuts, bee stings etc) has increased by 51% from 2001 to 2005 (see reference 59).

- Since the development of any disease results from a complex interplay between genetics, age, nutrition, socioeconomic factors and exposure to environmental chemicals (see reference 60) then one or more of these factors must be having an enhanced influence on disease incidence.

- **Nobody knows the precise relative importance** of these factors in disease development but it is accepted that environmental factors play an important role in the development of some diseases. One estimate is that 5-13% of human health problems are environmentally related (see reference 60).

- There is, however, considerable disagreement as to the relative importance of the Body Burden of chemicals in disease production with many people believing that **DEFINITIVE PROOF HAS YET TO BE PROVIDED** (see, the American Chemistry Council – Section 3, above).

- However, biomonitoring has revealed the presence of a mixture of toxic chemicals in the human body some of which have been shown to have **serious impacts on wildlife** populations of birds and mammals and fish (see, section 2, above). These chemicals include the persistent organic pollutants (POPs, Table 1) which have been shown to result in reproductive disorders, malformations and immune deficiency in wildlife at levels comparable to those in humans (see reference 60).

- There is particular concern regarding the many endocrine (hormone) disrupting chemicals (detailed in Table 1) that may affect foetal development, sperm count, onset of puberty and be linked to cancers sensitive to hormones. Even the unborn baby may be exposed to these via the mother's milk. These same chemicals have been shown to cause hormone disruption in wildlife and may therefore also affect humans similarly. Hormones normally act at very low levels so that even low levels of these artificial hormone mimics in the human body may have significant effects (see reference 60).

- It is also generally recognised that persistent organic pollutants (POPs) in Table 1, disrupt brain development in human foetuses and babies. PCBs, in particular, are linked to impaired learning and may affect movement and reflexes in children (see reference 60).

- Mixtures of azo dye food colourants have also been shown to increase hyperactivity in children (see Chapter 5 of IYL, Section 3), and sulphites have been included among the top 10 substances causing allergies.

- The quality of air inside houses may also be a source of health problems such as asthma, allergies, cancer in children (see reference 60) and adults. Chemicals found include PCBs, flame retardants and carcinogens, such as formaldehyde, from furnishings, paints and cleaners.

- There is evidence too that some childhood cancers are associated with exposure of the parents to pesticides and PAHs. These could be passed on to the foetus and baby via the mother's milk and induce mutations in these most susceptible and rapidly developing stages.

CONCLUSION

THERE'S NO SMOKE WITHOUT FIRE

REDUCE YOUR BODY BURDEN OF CHEMICALS

SECTION 5: AVOIDANCE AND REDUCTION OF BODY BURDEN OF CHEMICALS AND DETOX STRATEGIES

A number of basic steps can be followed to reduce your Body Burden of contaminants. The following are just **suggestions** that can be followed, a few at a time, depending on your situation, for example, if you or your children suffer from allergies and wish to reduce your chemical exposure.

TO AVOID PESTICIDES

- Buy some organic fruit and vegetables. It is **not necessary or possible to buy everything organic** and the most important fruit and vegetables to buy are listed at the end of Chapter 4 of IYL. Many fruits and vegetables that are peeled before eating have the lowest pesticide levels. Always wash fruit and vegetables in running water even if "ready washed" is written on the packaging.

- Many organic items are not regularly available or are too expensive in UK supermarkets in which case concentrate on buying organic **potatoes, bread, cereals, porridge** and **dairy,** which are usually available.

- Use pesticides / fungicides / herbicides around the home only if absolutely necessary. Do not follow popular gardening articles that may tell you to spray regularly. A few blighted potatoes are better than people breathing in or coming into contact with powerful toxins.

- Trim off excess fat from meat and skin from poultry as these may contain accumulated pesticides.

TO REDUCE ADDITIVES IN FOOD AND DRINK

- The easiest way of avoiding additives is to drink water or pure fruit juices and NOT soft drinks of any sort, buy fresh fruit and vegetables grown locally and read food labels to find out what chemical additives you are eating. **Refer to "Summary and how to reduce additives in your diet" at the end of Chapter 5 of IYL**.

- Unborn babies and young children with rapidly developing bodies will be **particularly vulnerable** to any harmful effects of additives.

- Trimming fat from meat and eating low fat dairy produce reduce dioxin intake.

TAKE CARE WITH PLASTICS

- Get rid of any polycarbonate baby bottles (usually marked with no.7 in triangle on bottom of bottles) as they may contain Bisphenol A (BPA).

- Never heat or microwave or wash in a dishwasher any plastic baby bottles.

- Use glass containers to heat baby food.

- Avoid canned food for babies and limit use in adults.

- Throw (recycle!) your plastic water bottles and do not reuse repeatedly.

- Do not store food for long periods in PVC wrap but use cellulose bags. Scrape off a thin layer of cheese stored in PVC before eating.

REDUCE THE CHEMICALS IN YOUR HEALTH AND BEAUTY PRODUCTS

- Sit down and read all the labels on your soaps, shampoos, toothpaste, exfoliants, body, hand and face creams, sunscreens, hair sprays and dyes, deodorants, shaving cream, lipstick, nail polish, perfumes etc. The list reads **like a chemical warfare mix** and not something that you expose your body to every day! See Table 1 of this Chapter for possible effects of these chemicals on your body.

- Maybe you suffer from allergies and maybe the chemicals in these products are making you worse?

- Ok, so you think that you cannot possibly go without any of these. However, what you can do is to note the main toxins present and try and buy products free of these (see references 61 and 62 for suppliers, and 63 for a safety review of cosmetics).

- From Table 1 you will see that there are **5 chemicals** in these products that are particularly important to try and eliminate:

1. Sodium lauryl sulphate (SLS or SDS) found in many liquid soaps (washing up liquids are particularly bad due to frequency of use) and shampoos, and causing dermatitis or allergic rhinitis (runny nose and sneezing).

2/3. The **phalates, such as DBP and DEHP,** and **parabens** (methyl-,ethyl-, propyl- and butyl- parabens), which are hormone disruptors. In the USA, the blood and urine of 20 teenage girls tested were found to contain parabens, as well as phalates in some (see reference 64).

4/5. The **polyethylene glycols (PEGs)** and **propylene glycol** that are irritants or contain carcinogens.

- As an example, you can buy "Simple Soap" without any of these 5 chemicals and also without fragrances which can also be a problem.

REDUCE CHEMICALS/IRRITANTS IN THE HOUSE

- It is very difficult to do this as the average house has many sources of contaminant chemicals in every day products.

- Have fun with the children and check out the toxic chemicals in a typical house (see reference 65).

- Buy more natural or environmentally safe cleaning agents (see reference 66) which are available for the toilet, washing up and for cleaning surfaces. Avoid "antibacterial" products (creating superbugs?) and always wear gloves when cleaning or washing up.

- Do not use insect sprays indoors.

- Use natural air fresheners like bunches of lavender in draws and cupboards.

- Avoid scented detergents/conditioners in the laundry.

- Use shoe cleaners outside with gloves on.

- Furnishings, carpets and mattresses will be treated with chemicals so try and find out what these are and decide if you want these in your home. Keep the rooms well aerated if possible and leave plastic covers in place for a while if possible. In particular, avoid flame retardants (PBDE) which are now banned in the EU.

- Store paints and cleaners well away from main living areas.

- If you are highly allergic, use house dust mite proof covers on bed linen.

- Vacuum clean regularly to reduce dust laden with household chemicals. Do not forget to vacuum the curtains.

- Use glass, stainless steel or cast iron cooking vessels rather than non-stick and Teflon-coated.

- Avoid dry cleaning clothes due to toxic solvents used.

DETOX, ESPECIALLY IF YOU ARE TRYING FOR A BABY

- The Body Burden of chemicals will continue to accumulate unless at least some of the above steps are followed to reduce the so-called **"Toxic Load"**. It makes sense to prevent further build up of contaminants which will subsequently be released into the body over many years.

- Normally, the body is extremely efficient at removing most toxins taken in but some, such as the dioxins and PCBs, accumulate in the fatty tissues. It has been estimated that some dioxins and PCBs can remain stored in the fat for 7-11 years or more (see reference 67).

- There is also a belief that the body can only accumulate a certain amount of contaminants and **above this maximal capacity** damage occurs resulting in allergies and ill health (see reference 68).

- The potential importance of reducing the Body Burden, especially for women planning a pregnancy, is illustrated by work showing **the transference of up to 69% of dioxins, as well as PCBs and other chemicals, from a mother's body into the fat of her milk during nursing of her baby** over a two year period (see reference 69).

- The Schecter study, however, is not scientifically significant as it only looked at one nursing mother and urgently needs repeating (see reference 69). There is also much debate as to whether these contaminants might cause harm to the baby.

- Finally, there are those who advocate active detox programmes to reduce the Body Burden as these have been shown to be successful. For example, following the collapse of the World Trade Centre, police, firemen, para-medics and labourers were exposed to high levels of PCBs and dioxins which accumulated at elevated levels in their bodies. A detoxification pro-gramme was undertaken and some significant reductions of pollutants were recorded which resulted in ad-verse health symptoms returning to normal (see reference 70).

- The value and safety, however, of such detox programmes are the subject of much debate. Some organisations are offering detox treatments which are not necessarily based upon sound and proven scientific and medical proof.

- The best approach is to reduce your Body Burden, as outlined above, making sure that you adopt a balanced diet (see Chapter 1 of IYL) to control your weight, and participate in a regular exercise programme (see Chapters 9-11 of IYL).

- Some additional references to detox methods, food and cosmetic additives as well as toxins in the environment are provided for those particularly concerned (see references 71-75).

The next book in the series is:

It's Your Life – Vitamins and Supplements For All Ages

For the complete guide to a healthy life:

It's Your Life: End the confusion from inconsistent health advice

Reference sources for conclusions

41. www.wwf.org.uk/filelibrary/pdf/biomonitoringresults.pdf

42. www.ewg.org/reports

43. Soni and colleagues, Food and Chemical Toxicology, Vol.43, pages 985-1015, 2005.

44. www.cosmeticsdatabase.co

45. Fruijtier-Polloth, Toxicology, Vol. 214, pp. 1-38, 2005, access at: Link-inghub.elsevier.com/retrieve/pii/S0300483X05002696

46. Bertazzi and colleagues, American Journal of Epidemiology Vol. 153, pages 1031-1044, 2001.

47. www.statcan.gc.ca/survey/household/measures/measures-mesures-eng.htm

48. www.biomonitoringinfo.org/new/20051128.html

49. www.wwf.org.uk/filelibrary/pdf/biomonitoringresults.pdf

50. www.ewg.org/sites/humantoxome/

51. http://cot.food.gov.uk/cotreports/cotwgreports/cocktail report

52. http://cot.food.gov.uk/cotreports/cotcomcocannreps/ cotcomcocrep2004

53. www.americanchemistry.com/s_acc/sec_acc_rcol.asp

54. http://assets.panda.org/downloads/12_pager_summary.pdf

55. Lau and colleagues, Toxicological Sciences, Vol. 90, pages 178-187, 2006.

56. www.food.gov.uk/news/newsarchive/2006/benzenesurvey

57. Laetz and colleagues, Environ. Health Perspect. Vol. 117, pages 348-353, 2009.

58. info.cancerresearchuk.org/cancerstats/types/testis/incidence

59. Sheikh and colleagues, J. Royal Society Medicine, Vol. 101, pages 139-143, 2008.

60. European Environment Agency Report No.10/2005, www.eea.europa.eu/publications/eea_report_2005_10

61. www.wen.org.uk with ref. 62 for names of suppliers of toxin-free cosmetics

62. www.devdelay.org/newsletter/articles/html/323-personal-care-products

63. www.ewg.org/Healthy-Home-Tips-01 for safety review of cosmetics

64. www.ewg.org/reports/teens

65. www.epa.gov/kidshometour

66. www.greenshop.co.uk

67. www.who.int/mediacentre/factsheets/fs225/en/index.html

68. Josef Krop, Healing the Planet, One Patient at a Time. A Primer in Environmental Medicine, 1997, (ISBN 0-9731945-0-2).

69. Schecter, Chemosphere, vol. 37, issue 9-12, pages 1807-1816, October 1998.

70. Dahlgren, Chemosphere, Volume 69, Issue 8, October 2007, Pages 1320-1325.

71. Wisner and colleagues, Treatment of children with detoxifica tion method developed by Hubbard, Proc. Amer. Public Health Assoc. National Conference, 1995.

72. Rapp, D.J. "Our Toxic World A Wakeup Call", 2004, see: www.drrapp.com/publications.htm

73. "Child-specific Exposure Factors Handbook", 2008, U.S.A. Environmental Protection Agency, Washington, USA.

74. "What's Really in Your Basket? An Easy Guide to Food additives and Cosmetics Ingredients, by Bill Statham, Summersdale Pub. 2007.

75. Richardson, A. "They Are What You Feed Them", 2006, see:

www.fabresearch.org/view_item.aspx?item_id=960